The Ultimate Guide to Achieving Flawless Skin

by

SANDRA BLAKE

Table of content

Introduction

Many individuals wish they could have skin that is flawless. However, achieving this objective might be difficult. Skin flaws may be caused by a variety of things, such as heredity, nutrition, lifestyle, and exposure to chemicals in the environment. The health and look of our skin may also be impacted by the aging process, hormonal changes, and certain medical problems.

Despite the difficulties, actions may be made to enhance the look of our skin and reach the coveted objective of flawless skin. The path to flawless skin may be a fulfilling one, from creating a reliable skincare regimen to altering one's lifestyle.

This manual's goal is to provide a thorough review of the procedures that may be used to acquire flawless skin. We'll go over the fundamentals of skincare, such as how crucial it is to clean, moisturize, and use sunscreen. In addition, we'll talk about how nutrition and lifestyle affect skin health and provide advice on how to treat common skin issues like acne, rosacea, and hyperpigmentation.

We will also explore the realm of cosmetic procedures and treatments, including the advantages and disadvantages of well-known procedures like chemical peels, microdermabrasion, and laser therapy. This book will provide you the knowledge and direction you need to attain the flawless skin you seek, whether you are just beginning your skincare journey or trying to improve your current regimen.

You will be well on your way to getting the healthy, vibrant, and flawless skin you have always desired if you heed the advice and suggestions included in this manual.

Chapter 1

Introduction to the Science of Skin Care

The biggest organ in your body, your skin is essential for keeping you hydrated, shielding you from the environment, and regulating body temperature. It's crucial to have a fundamental grasp of the science underlying skin care if you want to obtain flawless skin.

The three main layers of skin are the epidermis, dermis, and subcutaneous tissue. The skin's outermost layer, the epidermis, serves as a barrier to guard against environmental harm. Collagen, elastin, and other fibers that provide the skin structure and support are found in the dermis, which is the middle layer. The deepest layer, the subcutaneous tissue, serves as a cushion to guard against damage to the skin.

Sebaceous glands in the skin also secrete oil (sebum) to keep the skin moisturized. On the other hand, excessive sebum production may cause acne and clogged pores. The skin also has sweat glands that aid in controlling body temperature.

Wrinkles and age spots are two telltale symptoms of aging, and they may be brought on by aging, sun exposure, and other environmental factors that harm the skin. In addition to protecting the skin from additional harm, proper skin care may help lessen the look of aging.

In order to obtain flawless skin, it's crucial to develop a regular skin care routine and to have a basic grasp of the science of skin care. With the help of this manual, you may create a routine that is specific to your skin type and requirements. You may attain glowing, healthy skin that you'll be happy to display by following the instructions in this article.

Chapter 2

Understanding Your Skin Type

Understanding your skin type is one of the most crucial first steps to having flawless skin. Your skin type is influenced by a variety of factors, including heredity, hormone levels, and the environment, and it is subject to change over time. Normal, oily, dry, combination, and sensitive are the five primary varieties of skin.

Normal Skin: Normal skin is balanced, healthy-looking, and has few to no flaws. It is often devoid of blemishes and redness and is neither excessively dry nor overly greasy.

Oily Skin: Oily skin is characterized by excessive oil production, which causes blocked pores and a glossy complexion. Breakouts and blackheads are common with this skin type.

Dry Skin: Dry skin has a dull, flaky complexion since it doesn't produce enough natural oils. Redness, itching, and sensitivity are common with this type of skin.

Combination Skin: Combination skin is a combination of oily and dry skin, with oily patches (like the T-zone) and dry patches (like the cheeks).

Sensitive Skin: Sensitive skin is readily affected by cosmetics and external factors, which may result in redness, itching, and burning feelings. This skin type may also be more prone to allergies and breakouts.

Choosing the appropriate products and ingredients for your skin is made easier by knowing what type of skin you have. For instance, if you have oily skin, you should choose products that assist control oil production and clear clogged pores, but if you have dry skin, you should pick products that provide more moisture.

A simple patch test may be used to identify your skin type. Apply a toner to a tiny patch of skin after cleansing your face (such as the cheek or forehead). After waiting 15 minutes, check the skin. It will feel sticky and slippery if the skin is oily. It will feel tight and flaky if the skin is dry. It will feel elastic and velvety if the skin is healthy. To find out your general skin type, repeat the test on various facial features.

When you know what type of skin you have, you may create a skin care routine to assist you reach flawless skin. Beginning with the significance of washing, we'll go into each phase of a thorough skin care regimen in the following chapters.

Chapter 3

The Importance of a Skincare Routine

For flawless skin, you must establish a consistent skincare routine. The sun, wind, and pollution are just a few of the environmental factors that your skin is exposed to on a daily basis. These factors may harm your skin and induce the emergence of fine lines, wrinkles, and age spots.

Your skin may be protected from harm, the effects of aging can be delayed, and your skin can maintain its youthful appearance with the aid of a skincare routine. You may enhance the general health and look of your skin by adhering to a routine, which will give you a complexion that is radiant and young.

Knowing your skin type and using products designed particularly for it are the keys to a good skincare routine. For instance, if you have oily skin, you should choose products that assist control oil production and clear clogged pores, but if you have dry skin, you should pick products that provide more moisture.

The following actions have to be part of a standard skincare routine:

Cleanse: Cleaning is the first stage in a skincare routine, so it's crucial to choose a mild, non-irritating cleanser that will get rid of excess oil, makeup, and pollutants without drying out the skin.

Toning: Toning aids in restoring the pH balance of the skin, which might become off after washing. Additionally, a toner may aid in removing any last signs of pollutants or makeup.

Exfoliating: Exfoliating is a crucial component in a skincare routine since it aids in the removal of dead skin cells, which may block pores and result in outbreaks. Depending on your skin type and tolerance, you should exfoliate two to three times each week.

Treating entails using products to address certain skin issues, such as wrinkles, fine lines, or dark spots. Serums, masks, and eye creams are examples of such products. Moisturizing is crucial for all skin types because it keeps the skin hydrated and maintains its protective barrier. Apply moisturizer every morning and evening after cleaning and treating your skin with a moisturizer that is suitable for your skin type.

Even when it's overcast outside or you'll be spending most of your time inside, it's crucial to protect your skin from UV damage by applying a broad-spectrum sunscreen with an SPF of 30 or higher every day.

You may enhance the general health and look of your skin and achieve a glowing, young complexion by adhering to a regular skincare routine. The next chapter will go into further depth about each component of a skincare routine and provide advice on how to get the greatest results.

Chapter 4

Cleanse: The Foundation of a Skincare Routine

In a skincare routine, cleansing is the first and possibly most crucial step. It prepares your skin for the next stages by removing pollutants, makeup, and excess oil. It is the starting point for the remainder of your skincare routine. Cleansing also aids in pore clearing, which lessens the likelihood of breakouts and enhances the general health of your skin.

It is crucial to find a cleanser that is suitable for your skin type while making this decision. If you have oily skin, you may want to choose a foamy cleanser that helps regulate oil production and unclog pores, while if you have dry skin, you may want to select a creamy, moisturizing cleanser that won't deplete your skin of its natural oils. Selecting a mild, non-irritating cleanser that won't sting or sting your skin is crucial if you have sensitive skin.

Use the following methods to adequately cleanse your skin:

Apply warm water on your face. Your pores will become more open as a result of the warm water, which will make it simpler to eliminate contaminants.

Use your fingers to apply a little quantity of cleanser to your skin, then rub it in for approximately 30 seconds in a circular motion. Pay special attention to your T-zone (nasal bridge, chin, and forehead) and any other trouble spots.

Remove all remnants of the cleanser from your face by giving it a thorough rinse with warm water.

Dry off your face with a fresh towel.

Cleansing should be done twice a day, once in the morning and once at night, to remove pollutants and makeup. To make sure that all traces of makeup are eliminated, if you wear a lot of makeup, you may wish to use a makeup remover or cleansing oil before using your usual cleanser.

It's vital to choose a cleanser that is suitable for your skin type and to refrain from over-cleansing, which may deplete your skin of its natural oils and result in dryness, redness, and irritation. Additionally, over-cleansing may alter the pH balance of the skin, which can result in breakouts and other skin issues.

By thoroughly cleansing your skin, you remove pollutants, unclog pores, and get your skin ready for the rest of your skincare routine. This step cannot be neglected or ignored if you want to have healthy, beautiful skin.

Chapter 5

Tone: Balancing Your Skin's pH Level

The subsequent and crucial stage in a skincare routine is toning. Your skin's pH level might fall out of balance due to environmental factors like pollution and the use of harsh skincare products. Toning helps to restore that equilibrium. Dryness, sensitivity, and breakouts might result from an unbalanced pH level in your skin.

A toner helps to restore the pH balance of the skin, leaving it feeling moisturized and revitalized. Toners may also assist to tighten pores and get the skin ready for the next stages in your skincare routine by removing any residue from cleansers or makeup that may have been left behind.

It's crucial to pick a toner that is suitable for your skin type while making this decision. To assist control oil production and unclog pores, if you have oily skin, you may want to use a toner with astringent ingredients like witch hazel or tea tree oil. To assist add moisture to your skin, if you have dry skin, you may want to use a toner that has moisturizing ingredients like aloe vera or glycerin. A mild, alcohol-free toner that won't irritate or produce redness is crucial if you have sensitive skin.

The procedures for using a toner are as follows:

Apply a tiny quantity of toner on a cotton pad or your fingers after cleaning.

Gently sweep the toner over your face, giving special attention to your T-zone (forehead, nose, and chin) and any other trouble spots.

To let the toner sink into your skin, let it air-dry or give it a little pat with your hands.

As it helps to prepare the skin for the subsequent stages in your skincare routine, toning should be performed after cleaning and before moisturizing.

Along with selecting a toner that is suitable for your skin type, you should also avoid over-toning since this may deplete your skin's natural oils, resulting in dryness and irritation. Over-toning may also alter the pH balance of the skin, which can cause breakouts and other skin issues.

You can help your skin's pH level return to normal, get rid of pollutants and makeup, and get ready for the remainder of your skincare routine by toning your skin often. This stage should not be neglected or disregarded if you want healthy, beautiful skin.

Chapter 6

Exfoliate: Removing Dead Skin Cells

Exfoliation helps to eliminate dead skin cells and expose new, healthy skin, making it a crucial element in any skincare regimen. In addition to preventing breakouts and congested pores, regular exfoliation helps to keep your skin appearing young and vibrant.

The accumulation of dead skin cells on the skin's surface may make it seem dull and feel rough. Your skin will seem softer, more luminous, and smoother after exfoliating, which helps to eliminate these dead skin cells.

Exfoliants come in two varieties: chemical and physical. While chemical exfoliants employ enzymes or acids to breakdown and remove the dead skin cells, physical exfoliants use tiny particles or bristles to physically brush away dead skin cells.

Alpha-hydroxy acids (AHAs) and beta-hydroxy acids are examples of chemical exfoliants, whereas sponges, brushes, and scrubs are examples of physical exfoliants (BHAs). While chemical exfoliants are best for those with sensitive or easily irritated skin, physical exfoliants are best for people with tough, rough skin.

Follow these instructions to use an exfoliant:

Remove any makeup or pollutants from your face using a cleanser.

Carefully avoid the eye region when you apply a little quantity of exfoliant to your hands and gently massage it into your skin in a circular motion.

For the prescribed duration, which is often 1-2 minutes, leave the exfoliant on.

Use a clean towel to gently wipe your skin dry after rinsing the exfoliant off with warm water.

It's crucial to keep in mind that exfoliating more often than once or twice a week might lead to sensitivity, dryness, and irritation. Additionally, it's crucial to choose an exfoliant suitable for your skin type since certain exfoliants might be too harsh for skin that's already sensitive.

Exfoliating is a crucial part of any skincare routine since it may assist to reveal skin that is lighter, smoother, and more vibrant. You may avoid breakouts, blocked pores, and dull, lifeless skin by exfoliating dead skin cells. Exfoliation should not be ignored or neglected since it may help you obtain healthy, youthful-looking skin.

Chapter 7

Treat: Addressing Specific Skin Concerns

Treatment with certain products may assist to target specific skin concerns including fine lines, wrinkles, dark spots, and acne in addition to cleansing, toning, and exfoliating your skin. Serums, facial oils, eye creams, and masks are just a few of the treatments that are accessible.

Serums are thin, quickly absorbed liquids that are intended to deliver potent active ingredients deep into the skin. They may be used to treat a range of skin issues, such as wrinkles, dark spots, and uneven skin tone.

Because they moisturize, feed, and refresh the skin, face oils are ideal for those with dry or older skin. To give your skin more moisture and nutrition, you may use face oils alone or in combination with moisturizers.

The sensitive skin around the eyes, which is often the first place to exhibit symptoms of aging, is addressed with eye lotions that are particularly made for this area. Eye creams may assist in lessening the visibility of fine lines, wrinkles, and dark circles, giving your eyes a more young and bright appearance.

Using masks is an excellent approach to hydrate and nourish your skin. They may be used monthly or biweekly to deal with certain skin issues and provide a thorough cleanse. There are many different types of masks, including clay, sheet, and hydrogel masks.

Since certain treatments may be too potent for everyday use or may induce sensitivity if taken too often, it is crucial to adhere to the stated usage guidelines while utilizing them. Additionally, it is crucial to choose treatments that are suitable for your skin type since some might be too harsh for skin that is already sensitive.

You may address certain skin issues and enhance the look and health of your skin overall by including treatments into your skincare routine. There is a treatment that may help you reach your skin objectives, whether you want to lessen the appearance of fine lines and wrinkles, lighten dark spots, or soothe acne-prone skin.

Chapter 8

Moisturize: Hydrating Your Skin

In order to keep the skin hydrated and prevent moisture loss, moisturizing is a crucial component in any skincare routine. Your skin will feel soft, smooth, and luminous after moisturizing regularly, which may help prevent dryness, flakiness, and premature aging.

Moisturizers come in two varieties: water-based and oil-based. Because they provide a deep, nourishing hydration, oil-based moisturizers are ideal for those with dry or aged skin. Because they are lighter and less greasy, water-based moisturizers are best for those with oily or mixed skin.

Follow these instructions to apply a moisturizer:

Remove any makeup or pollutants from your face using a cleanser.

To balance the pH of your skin, tone it.

Use your fingers to apply a little quantity of moisturizer, then gently massage it into your skin in an upward and outward motion.

Before wearing any makeup or sunscreen, give the moisturizer time to seep into your skin.

As some moisturizers might be too thick for oily skin or too light for dry skin, it is crucial to choose a moisturizer that is suitable for your skin type. In order to protect your skin from UV damage, it is also crucial to apply a moisturizer with SPF protection.

In order to moisturize and preserve the skin, moisturizing is a crucial component in any skincare routine. By properly hydrating your skin, you may avoid dryness, flakiness, and early aging and attain healthy, vibrant skin. It's vital to include moisturizing in your daily skincare routine whether you have dry, oily, or mixed skin.

Chapter 9

The Role of Sunscreen in Flawless Skin

Sunscreen is one of the most important products in your skincare routine, as it helps to protect your skin from harmful UV rays that can cause sunburn, skin aging, and skin cancer. Regular use of sunscreen can help to prevent premature aging, dark spots, and other signs of sun damage, leaving your skin looking youthful and radiant.

Chemical and physical sunscreens are the two varieties. Active chemicals in chemical sunscreens absorb UV radiation and transform them into heat, which is subsequently expelled from the skin. Physical sunscreens contain active ingredients that physically block UV rays from penetrating the skin.

To use sunscreen, follow these steps:

- Cleanse your face to remove any makeup or impurities.

- To balance the pH of your skin, tone it.

- Apply a generous amount of sunscreen to your face and neck, making sure to cover all exposed areas.

- Every two hours, or after swimming or perspiring, reapply.It is important to choose a sunscreen that is appropriate for your skin type, as some sunscreens can be too heavy for oily skin or too light for dry skin. Additionally, it is important to choose a sunscreen with a high SPF, as this will provide maximum protection from UV rays.

Sunscreen is a critical component of a skincare routine, as it helps to protect your skin from harmful UV rays that can cause sunburn, skin aging, and skin cancer. By using a high-quality sunscreen daily, you can help to prevent premature aging, dark spots, and other signs of sun damage, and achieve flawless, radiant skin.

Chapter 10

The Benefits of Antioxidants for the Skin

Antioxidants are compounds that help to protect the skin from damage caused by free radicals, which are unstable molecules that can cause oxidative stress and contribute to aging and disease. Antioxidants work by neutralizing free radicals and protecting the skin from damage, which can result in a more youthful and radiant complexion.

There are many different types of antioxidants, including vitamins C and E, beta-carotene, and resveratrol. These antioxidants can be found in a variety of skincare products, such as serums, creams, and masks, and can provide a range of benefits for the skin.

Some of the benefits of antioxidants for the skin include:

Protection against oxidative stress: Antioxidants help to protect the skin from damage caused by free radicals, which can contribute to aging and disease.

Brightening of the skin: Antioxidants can help to brighten the skin and reduce the appearance of dark spots and other discoloration.

Reduction of fine lines and wrinkles: Antioxidants can help to reduce the appearance of fine lines and wrinkles, resulting in a more youthful complexion.

Improved skin texture: Antioxidants can help to improve the texture of the skin, making it feel softer and smoother.

To incorporate antioxidants into your skincare routine, you can use an antioxidant-rich serum or cream, or incorporate antioxidant-rich foods into your diet, such as berries, dark leafy greens, and nuts.

The benefits of antioxidants for the skin are numerous, and incorporating these powerful compounds into your skincare routine can help to protect your skin from damage, reduce the appearance of aging, and achieve a more youthful and radiant complexion. Whether you choose to use topical products or incorporate antioxidant-rich foods into your diet, incorporating antioxidants into your skincare routine is an important step towards achieving flawless skin.

Chapter 11

Essential Oils for Skincare: Choosing the Right Ones

Essential oils have been used for centuries for their therapeutic properties, and are now becoming increasingly popular as a natural solution for skin care. These highly concentrated plant extracts contain active compounds that can provide a range of benefits for the skin, from reducing inflammation to promoting skin hydration.

However, it is important to choose the right essential oils for your skin type, as some oils can be too strong or irritating for sensitive skin. Here are some of the most commonly used essential oils for skincare, and their benefits:

Lavender Oil: Lavender oil is known for its calming and soothing properties, and is often used to treat skin irritations, such as eczema and psoriasis.

Tea Tree Oil: Tea tree oil is a natural antiseptic that can help to kill bacteria and reduce inflammation, making it ideal for use on acne-prone skin.

Rosehip Oil: Rosehip oil is high in antioxidants and fatty acids, making it ideal for use on mature or aging skin. It can help to reduce the appearance of fine lines and wrinkles, and promote skin hydration.

Frankincense Oil: Frankincense oil is known for its anti-inflammatory properties, and can help to improve the appearance of scars and other skin imperfections.

Jojoba Oil: Jojoba oil is a light and non-greasy oil that is ideal for use on all skin types, including oily skin. It can help to regulate sebum production and promote skin hydration.

To use essential oils in your skincare routine, you can add a few drops to your moisturizer, or use them in a DIY face mask. It is also important to dilute essential oils with a carrier oil, such as jojoba oil or coconut oil, before applying to the skin, as they can be very concentrated and irritating to the skin.

Incorporating essential oils into your skincare routine can provide a range of benefits for your skin, from reducing inflammation to promoting skin hydration. However, it is important to choose the right essential oils for your skin type, and to use them safely and responsibly, to ensure that you achieve the best results.

Chapter 12

Eating for Flawless Skin: A Guide to a Healthy Diet

In terms of skin health and attractiveness, your food is quite important. In fact, what you eat can either enhance or detract from your skin's radiance and overall health. A diet that is rich in nutrients, vitamins, and minerals can help to improve the look and feel of your skin, while a diet that is high in processed foods, sugar, and unhealthy fats can lead to dull, dry, and blemished skin.

Here are some key components of a diet for flawless skin:

Hydration: Staying hydrated is essential for maintaining healthy skin. Aim to drink at least eight glasses of water a day, and consider adding more water-rich foods, such as fruits and vegetables, to your diet.

Antioxidants: Antioxidants help to protect your skin from damage caused by free radicals, which can lead to premature aging and other skin problems. Berries, dark chocolate, and green tea are examples of foods that are rich in antioxidants.

Omega-3 Fatty Acids: Omega-3 fatty acids are essential for maintaining healthy skin, as they help to reduce inflammation and promote skin hydration. Omega-3 fatty acids may be found in salmon, flaxseeds, and walnuts.

Vitamins and Minerals: Vitamins and minerals, such as Vitamin A, Vitamin C, and Zinc, play an important role in skin health, and can help to improve the appearance of your skin. Good sources of these vitamins and minerals include sweet potatoes, bell peppers, and oysters.

Fiber: A diet that is high in fiber can help to support the health of your skin by promoting digestive health and reducing inflammation. Good sources of fiber include whole grains, legumes, and fruits and vegetables.

In addition to these key components, it is also important to limit or avoid certain foods that can have a negative impact on your skin, such as sugar, dairy, and processed foods.

By incorporating these key components into your diet, you can help to ensure that your skin looks and feels its best. A healthy diet, combined with a consistent skincare routine, can help you to achieve and maintain flawless skin.

Chapter 13

Sleep and Stress Management for Better Skin

Getting enough sleep and managing stress are critical components of a healthy skin routine. Not only do these factors impact your overall health and well-being, but they can also have a significant impact on the appearance of your skin.

Sleep:

Sleep is essential for skin health as it provides your body with the time it needs to repair and regenerate itself, including your skin. During sleep, your skin works to repair damage from the day and produce collagen, which helps to maintain the skin's elasticity and reduce the appearance of fine lines and wrinkles. Aim to get at least 7-9 hours of sleep each night, and make sure to create a sleep environment that is conducive to rest, such as keeping your bedroom cool, dark, and quiet.

Stress Management:

Stress can take a toll on your skin, causing problems such as breakouts, dry skin, and wrinkles. To reduce the impact of stress on your skin, it is important to find ways to manage stress in your life. This can include exercise, yoga, meditation, and spending time in nature. You can also incorporate stress-reducing activities into your skincare routine, such as taking a relaxing bath or using aromatherapy.

In addition, it is important to avoid stress-inducing behaviors, such as overeating or smoking, as these can have a negative impact on your skin.

By prioritizing sleep and stress management, you can help to ensure that your skin looks and feels its best. A healthy sleep routine and effective stress management strategies can help you to achieve and maintain flawless skin, both inside and out.

Chapter 14

How to Pick Your Ideal Skincare Products

With so many skincare products on the market, choosing the right ones for your skin type can be overwhelming. To find the best products for your skin, it is important to understand your skin type and any specific skin concerns you may have.

Consider Your Skin Type:

The first step in choosing the right skincare products is to identify your skin type. Common skin types include oily, dry, combination, sensitive, and mature. Once you have identified your skin type, you can look for products that are specifically designed for your skin. For example, if you have oily skin, look for products that are oil-free and non-comedogenic, which will help to control oil production and prevent breakouts.

Evaluate Ingredients:

Pay close attention to the ingredients list while selecting skincare products. Look for products that contain ingredients that are known to benefit your skin type and address any specific skin concerns you may have. For example, if you have sensitive skin, look for products that contain soothing ingredients like aloe vera and chamomile. If you have fine lines and wrinkles, look for products that contain retinoids or hyaluronic acid, which can help to improve skin texture and reduce the appearance of wrinkles.

Do Your Research:

Investigate your options carefully before purchasing a new skincare item. Read reviews from other users, and pay attention to any potential side effects or skin reactions. You can also consult with a dermatologist or skincare professional for recommendations and advice.

Trying Before You Buy:

When possible, try a small sample of a product before making a full purchase. This will give you an opportunity to see how your skin reacts to the product and determine if it is the right choice for you.

By considering your skin type, evaluating ingredients, doing your research, and trying before you buy, you can choose the right skincare products for your skin and achieve your best, most flawless complexion.

Chapter 15

Skincare Mistakes to Avoid

While a good skincare routine can have many benefits for your skin, making certain mistakes can actually do more harm than good. Here are some common skincare mistakes to avoid:

Over-Exfoliating:

Exfoliating is an important part of any skincare routine, but over-exfoliating can damage your skin. Over-exfoliating can lead to skin irritation, dryness, and even breakouts. It is important to stick to a regular exfoliating schedule, and to choose gentle exfoliants that are suitable for your skin type.

Using Dirty Tools:

Using dirty tools, such as makeup brushes or facial sponges, can introduce bacteria and other contaminants onto your skin. This can lead to breakouts and skin infections. It is important to regularly clean and sanitize your skincare tools to avoid this issue.

Skipping Sunscreen:

Sunscreen is an essential part of any skincare routine, as it helps to protect your skin from harmful UV rays. Skipping sunscreen can lead to sunburns, premature aging, and an increased risk of skin cancer. Make sure to use a broad-spectrum sunscreen with at least SPF 30 every day, regardless of the weather.

Using Harsh Products:

Using harsh products, such as alcohol-based toners or products with high concentrations of active ingredients, can strip your skin of its natural oils and cause irritation. It is important to choose gentle, non-irritating products that are suitable for your skin type.

Neglecting Hydration:

Drinking plenty of water and using a good moisturizer are important for keeping your skin hydrated. Neglecting hydration can lead to dry, flaky skin and can even make other skin concerns, such as fine lines and wrinkles, more noticeable.

By avoiding these common skincare mistakes, you can help to protect your skin and achieve your best, most flawless complexion.

Chapter 16

The Power of Natural Skincare Ingredients

When it comes to achieving flawless skin, many people turn to natural skincare ingredients for their effectiveness and gentleness. Here are some of the most powerful natural ingredients and how they can benefit your skin:

Aloe Vera:

Aloe vera is a popular natural ingredient that has been used for centuries to soothe and hydrate the skin. It is a rich source of vitamins, minerals, and antioxidants, and is known for its ability to help heal sunburns, reduce redness and inflammation, and improve skin elasticity.

Honey:

Honey is a natural humectant that attracts and retains moisture in the skin. It is also a natural antibacterial agent, which makes it a great choice for treating acne-prone skin. Honey can also help to soothe and calm irritated skin, and can even improve the appearance of fine lines and wrinkles.

Coconut Oil:

Coconut oil is a versatile skincare ingredient that is known for its moisturizing properties. It is rich in fatty acids, vitamins, and antioxidants, which help to hydrate, nourish, and protect the skin. Coconut oil can also be used as a makeup remover, and can even be used to treat skin conditions such as eczema and psoriasis.

Green Tea:

Green tea is a natural ingredient that is rich in antioxidants and anti-inflammatory compounds. It can help to protect the skin from damage caused by free radicals, and can also help to improve the appearance of fine lines and wrinkles. Green tea can also help to soothe and calm irritated skin, and can even help to reduce redness and puffiness.

Lavender:

Lavender is a natural ingredient that is known for its soothing and calming properties. It can help to reduce redness and inflammation, and can even help to improve the appearance of fine lines and wrinkles. Lavender can also help to hydrate and nourish the skin, and can even be used to treat skin conditions such as acne and eczema.

By incorporating natural skincare ingredients into your routine, you can enjoy the many benefits that they have to offer, while avoiding harsh chemicals and artificial ingredients. Whether you choose to use these ingredients in their pure form, or to look for products that contain them, they can help you to achieve a more beautiful, healthy complexion.

Chapter 17

Skincare on a Budget: Affordable Options for Flawless Skin

Having a healthy, glowing complexion doesn't have to be expensive. There are many affordable skincare options that can help you achieve flawless skin, regardless of your budget. Here are some tips for maintaining a budget-friendly skincare routine:

Look for Multi-Purpose Products: Instead of buying a separate cleanser, toner, and moisturizer, look for products that can do multiple jobs. This will help you save money and simplify your routine.

Use Natural Ingredients: Many natural ingredients, such as coconut oil, honey, and aloe vera, can be used on their own to cleanse, hydrate, and nourish your skin. These ingredients are often more affordable than commercial skincare products, and they're gentle and effective.

Make Your Own Products: There are many DIY skincare recipes that you can make at home using natural ingredients. Not only are these recipes affordable, but they're also customizable, so you can tailor them to your specific skin needs.

Prioritize Sun Protection: Sunscreen is an essential part of a healthy skincare routine, and it's also one of the most affordable options. Look for a broad-spectrum sunscreen with an SPF of at least 30, and apply it every day, even on cloudy days.

Shop Sales and Coupons: Keep an eye out for sales and coupons when shopping for skincare products. Many stores offer discounts on popular skincare brands, and you can also find coupons online.

Invest in High-Quality Products: While it's important to stick to a budget, it's also important to invest in high-quality skincare products that are right for your skin. Choose products that are formulated with natural ingredients and free of harmful chemicals, and look for those that address your specific skin concerns.

By following these tips, you can keep your skincare routine budget-friendly while still achieving the flawless skin you desire. Don't be afraid to experiment with different products and ingredients, and remember that the most important part of a skincare routine is consistency and commitment.

Chapter 18

Maintaining Flawless Skin: Staying on Track and Celebrating Your Journey

Achieving flawless skin is not a one-time event, but rather a lifelong journey. By following a consistent skincare routine, eating a healthy diet, getting enough sleep, and managing stress, you can maintain healthy, glowing skin for years to come. Here are some tips for staying on track and celebrating your journey to flawless skin:

Keep a Skincare Diary: Keeping a diary of your skincare routine can help you stay accountable and track your progress. Write down what products you use, when you use them, and how your skin is feeling. This can help you identify any patterns or changes in your skin and make adjustments to your routine as needed.

Celebrate Small Wins: Celebrating your small wins along the way can help keep you motivated and positive about your journey. Whether it's the disappearance of a blemish, the improvement of your skin texture, or just a general feeling of confidence, acknowledge and celebrate these wins.

Find a Support System: Having a support system of friends or family members who also care about their skincare can help keep you accountable and motivated. Share your skincare journey with others, and look for ways to support each other.

Stay Committed: Consistency is key when it comes to maintaining flawless skin. Make a commitment to stick to your skincare routine every day, and don't be discouraged if you have setbacks along the way. Just keep pushing forward and reminding yourself of your goals.

Take Care of Yourself: In addition to following a consistent skincare routine, make sure you're taking care of yourself in other ways. Get enough sleep, eat a healthy diet, manage stress, and make time for self-care and relaxation.

Embrace Your Journey: Remember that your journey to flawless skin is unique to you, and that's okay. Embrace your individual journey, and don't compare yourself to others. Celebrate your accomplishments and take pleasure in the journey. By following these tips, you can stay on track and celebrate your journey to flawless skin. Remember that this is a lifelong journey, and that it's okay to have setbacks along the way. Just stay committed to your skincare routine, and remember that the journey is just as important as the destination.

www.ingramcontent.com/pod-product-compliance
Lightning Source LLC
Chambersburg PA
CBHW081833250726
48657CB00019B/3503